Ramen Recipe Book for Beginners

Quick and Easy Ramen Collection Recipes

Jonathan Rees

© Copyright 2020 - All rights reserved.

The content contained within this book may not be reproduced, duplicated or transmitted without direct written permission from the author or the publisher.

Under no circumstances will any blame or legal responsibility be held against the publisher, or author, for any damages, reparation, or monetary loss due to the information contained within this book. Either directly or indirectly.

Legal Notice:

This book is copyright protected. This book is only for personal use. You cannot amend, distribute, sell, use, quote or paraphrase any part, or the content within this book, without the consent of the author or publisher.

Disclaimer Notice:

Please note the information contained within this document is for educational and entertainment purposes only. All effort has been executed to present accurate, up to date, and reliable, complete information. No warranties of any kind are declared or implied. Readers acknowledge that the author is not engaging in the rendering of legal, financial, medical or professional advice. The content within this book has been derived from various sources. Please consult a licensed professional before attempting any techniques outlined in this book.

By reading this document, the reader agrees that under no circumstances is the author responsible for any losses, direct or indirect, which are incurred as a result of the use of information contained within this document, including, but not limited to, — errors, omissions, or inaccuracies.

Table of Contents

Ramen noodles a basic recipe 7

Bami Goreng 10

Broccoli Shrimp Ramen 12

Burger bowl 14

Cheeseburger bowl 16

Chicken Teriyaki 18

Chinese cabbage ramen with turkey 20

Creamy ramen 22

Curry coconut ramen 24

Curry ramen 26

Dan Dan Ramen 29

English Breakfast 33

Peanut Curry Ramen 35

Peanut ramen with sesame seeds 37

Refreshing Chicken Ramen 39

Prawn ramen 41

Shrimp Garlic Ramen 44

Fried ramen 47

Grilled chicken ramen 50

Vegetable ramen 52

Vegetable beef ramen 55

All sorts of green 57

Guacamole bowl 59

Ramen with meatballs 62

Black pepper 63

Chicken ramen with lime 65

Hoisin ramen 67

Ginger Chicken Ramen 69

Ginger beef ramen 71

Ginger-lemongrass ramen 74

Scallop and asparagus ramen 76

Cheese ramen 78

Garlic ramen 81

Garlic Sesame Ramen 83

Coconut ramen 85

Salmon ramen 89

Salmon and Brussels sprouts bowl 92

Corn miso ramen 95

Matcha ramen (vegan) 99

Seafood ramen 102

Minute ramen 105

Ramen noodles a basic recipe

for 3 servings

for 40 minutes

ingredients

50 grams of water, cold

50 grams of water, warm

200 grams of wheat flour type 550

2 teaspoons of baked soda

preparation

1. Dissolve 2 teaspoons of baked soda in 100 grams of warm water. Then put this mixture in a large bowl along with the cold water and add the flour. Use the dough hook of a hand mixer to stir the contents of the bowl until crumbly dough is formed.

2. Place the dough on a work surface and knead it with your hands for five minutes to make smooth and chewy dough. Wrap this in plastic wrap and let it sit at room temperature for 20 minutes.

3. Take the dough out of the cling film and knead it by hand for another five minutes. Then wrap it again in foil and let it sit in the refrigerator for another hour.

4. Divide the dough into 3 portions and roll it out thinly on a floured work surface. Ideally, the dough should be about 1 millimeter thick. Then use a sharp knife to cut it into very thin strips. Alternatively, you can also use a machine with a spaghetti attachment. Flour the work surface over and over during this step.

5. Spread the finished noodles on a large surface, dust them with flour and loosen them up again. You can also prepare the ramen noodles and use them later - it's okay if they dry out a little.

6. Put the pasta in a large saucepan with plenty of water to cook. Cook the pasta in it for about 2 to 3 minutes and drain immediately. Then rinse the ramen directly with cold water to pause the cooking process, rinse off the excess starch, and prevent the ramen from sticking together.

INFO

You can easily make your own baked soda. To do this, put 4 packets of baking powder on a baking sheet, which you line up with baking paper beforehand. Then put the whole thing in the oven for 1 hour at 130 ° to 150 ° degrees. Then let the baked soda cool and transfer it to storage jars for storage.

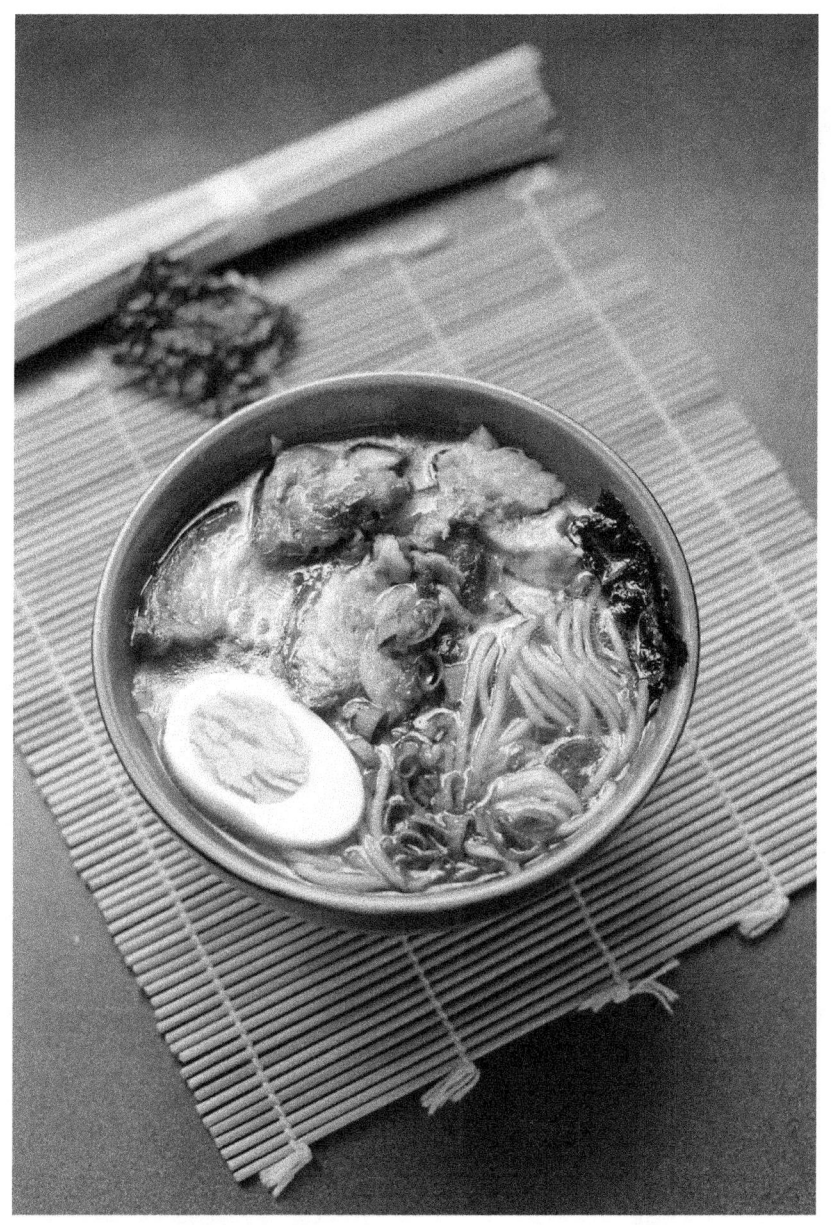

Bami Goreng

for 3 servings

for 30 minutes

ingredients

100 grams of sugar snap peas

125 grams of shrimp

125 grams of ramen

3 handfuls of mung bean sprouts

½ chili, cut into rings

1 piece of ginger, pressed

1 large carrot, cut into sticks

1 large onion, diced

2 half chicken breasts diced

2 cloves of garlic, pressed

4 large leaves of white cabbage cut into small pieces Chili sauce or sambal oelek Ketjap Manis

Garlic pepper

Soy sauce, dark

preparation

1   Cook the ramen al dente, then drain and drain well.

2   Heat some oil in a wok and sear the chicken in it. Then add the prawns and season the contents of the wok with the garlic pepper. Add the sugar snap peas and cook covered for about 10 minutes.

3   Add the beans, chili, ginger, carrot, garlic, ramen and white cabbage and let cook, covered, for another 5 minutes.

4   Season the dish with ketjap manis, garlic pepper, sambal oelek and the soy sauce and serve immediately.

Broccoli Shrimp Ramen

for 2 servings

for 30 minutes

ingredients

200 grams of shrimp

240 grams of ramen

400 milliliters of poultry broth

½ broccoli

2 eggs

2 spring onions

pepper

salt

preparation

1   Wash the broccoli and spring onions thoroughly. Divide the broccoli into florets and finely chop the spring onions.

2   Boil the ramen al dente, then drain them and let them cool in ice water. Meanwhile, cook the eggs until they are waxy for 6 minutes, frighten them off, peel them and then cut them in half.

3   Boil the broth and season with salt and pepper. Add the broccoli florets and let them cook in the broth for about 4 minutes.

4   Add the spring onions and ramen to the broth and let them cook too.

5   Spread the ramen, broccoli and spring onions on bowls, pour the broth over them and garnish the dish with the halved eggs and shrimp.

Burger bowl

for 4 servings

for 40 minutes

ingredients

100 grams of ramen

500 grams of pan-frozen vegetables

500 grams of ground beef

75 milliliters stir fry sauce

375 milliliters of water

preparation

1   Heat some oil in a pan over medium heat and fry the beef in it. Add the vegetables, sauce and water and bring everything to a boil while stirring.

2   Reduce the heat of the pan and let the pan's contents cook for about 5 minutes, stirring occasionally, until the vegetables are crispy or tender.

3   Break the ramen and add them to the pan. Stir them in well, cover the pan and cook the dish for another 5 to 8 minutes,

stirring occasionally, until the sauce has thickened and the ramen is soft. Divide the ramen in bowls and serve immediately.

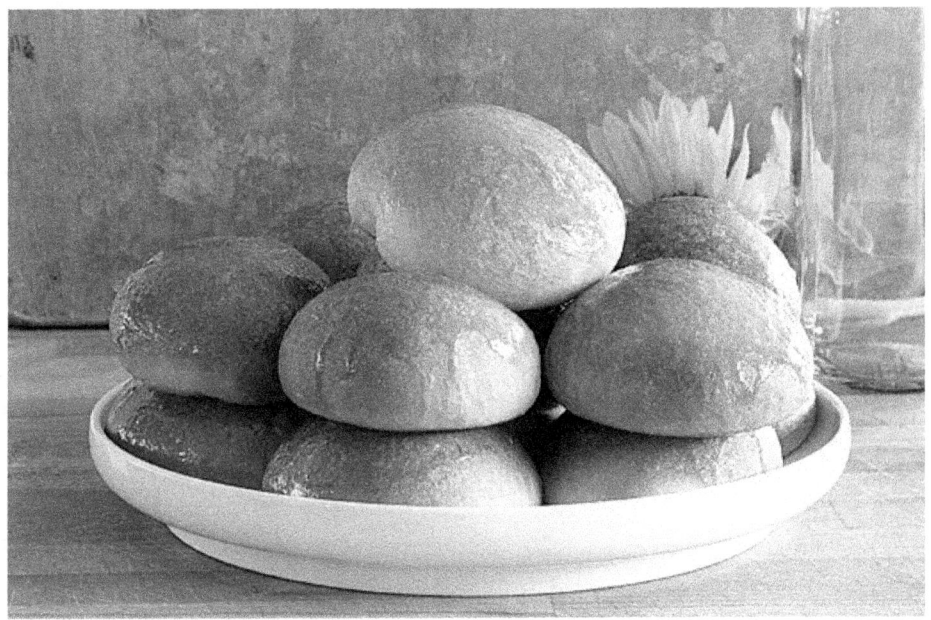

Cheeseburger bowl

    for 6 servings

for 40 minutes

easily

ingredients

100 grams of cheesy bread, diced

100 grams of onions, chopped

150 grams of ramen

425 grams of canned tomato cubes

500 grams of ground beef

75 milliliters of ketchup

230 milliliters of tomato sauce

2 teaspoons of mustard

Dill pickles

Lettuce, torn

Tomatoes, chopped

preparation

1   Preheat the oven to 175 degrees.

2   Grease a 22-centimeter square baking dish. Put the beef and onions in the baking dish and then cook them in the oven at 165 degrees until the meat turns brown.

3   Break the ramen into four pieces of relatively equal length and place them in the baking dish along with the ketchup, mustard, tomatoes and tomato sauce.

4   Cover the baking dish and bake for 25 minutes. Then add the bread cubes and bake for another five minutes until the cheese melts.

5   Serve the dish garnished with the dill pickles, the lettuce and the chopped tomatoes.

Chicken Teriyaki

for 2 servings

Less than 30 minutes
easily

ingredients

60 grams of sugar snap peas

200 grams of chicken breast

400 grams of ramen

800 milliliters of chicken stock

1 teaspoon sugar, brown

1 tablespoon of rapeseed oil

6 tablespoons of mirin

6 tablespoons of sake

6 tablespoons of soy sauce

¼ of a leek, white section
1 egg, size M
salt

preparation

1   Boil the stock in a wide saucepan, let it boil uncovered on high heat for 10 minutes so that the liquid is reduced to about 600 milliliters. Heat the mirin, sake, soy sauce and sugar in a small saucepan and let it simmer for about 10 minutes until a s thick teriyaki sauce is formed.

2   Heat water in a saucepan and cook the eggs in it for 6 minutes until they become waxy. Then rinse them with cold water, peel them, and let them cool in ice water. Halve the eggs lengthways.

3   Wash the leeks, clean them thoroughly and cut them into thin rings. Wash and clean the sugar snap peas, then blanch them in boiling salted water for 1 minute. Pour off the water and soak the sugar snap peas in ice water for 2 minutes. Drain the water again and set the sugar snap peas aside for now.

4   Pat the chicken breast dry with a paper towel. Heat some oil in a pan and fry the meat on medium heat for about 4 to 5 minutes on each side. Then glaze them with 1 tablespoon of the teriyaki sauce. Then cut the chicken breast pieces into 5-millimeter-thick strips.

5   Cook the ramen, drain and drain well. Spread the remaining teriyaki sauce on the bowls and pour the hot stock over them. Then add the ramen and use a fork to twist them up in a spiral. Then add the egg, chicken, leek, and snow peas and serve immediately.

Chinese cabbage ramen with turkey

for 4 servings

for 30 minutes

easily

ingredients

200 grams of ramen

400 grams of turkey breast fillet

600 grams of Chinese cabbage, cut into strips

1 teaspoon of sugar

1 tablespoon cornstarch

4 tablespoons of oil

4 tablespoons of soy sauce

1 clove of garlic, diced

1 onion, diced

3 carrots, halved, sliced

pepper

salt

preparation

1 Cook the ramen al dente, then drain and drain well. Mix them with 1 tablespoon of oil to avoid sticking together. Pat the meat dry with a paper towel and cut it into cubes. Turn it in cornstarch until it is completely covered.

2   Heat 3 tablespoons of oil in a wok and fry the meat until golden brown on

all sides. Season it with the pepper and salt and remove it from the

pan. Cover and fry the carrots and onions in the roasting tray for about 5 minutes. Then add the Chinese cabbage and cook it for 10 minutes, turning occasionally. If necessary, add some liquid to the pan.

3   Add all the other ingredients to the wok and stir them in well. Season the dish with pepper, soy sauce and sugar and serve immediately.

Creamy ramen

for 2 servings

Less than 30 minutes

easily

ingredients

100 grams of ramen

40 milliliters of milk

300 milliliters of water

2 tablespoons of butter

Your choice of spices

preparation

1. Boil the water in a small saucepan. Then add the ramen to the water and cook them for about 3 minutes, stirring occasionally, until they take on a soft consistency. Drain the water and let the ramen drain well.

2. Put the ramen back in the empty saucepan and add the butter and

milk. Season the sauce with your choice of spices. Cook the whole thing over low heat until the butter is completely melted and the ramen is coated with the creamy sauce.

3   Put the ramen in bowls and serve immediately.

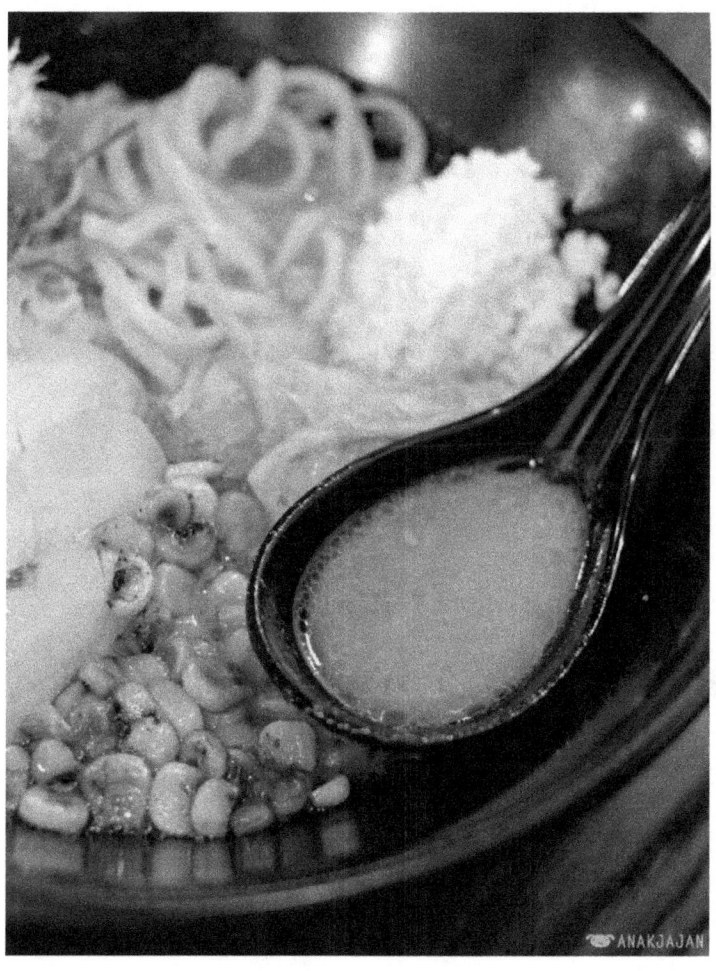

Curry coconut ramen

for 4 servings

less than 30 minutes

easily

ingredients

125 grams of peanut butter

200 grams of ramen

500 grams of shrimp, peeled, deveined, cooked

75 milliliters of coconut milk

¼ teaspoon pepper flakes, red

2 tablespoons of lime juice, fresh

2 cucumbers

4 spring onions

Lime wedges

preparation

1. Wash the spring onions and cucumbers and cut both into small pieces.

2 Boil 600 milliliters of water in a large saucepan. Break the ramen into quarters and add them to the boiling water. Cover the pot, remove it from the stove, and let the ramen steep for about 5 minutes.

3 In a large bowl, stir together the peanut butter, coconut milk and pepper flakes.

4 Let the ramen drain well and add them to the dressing bowl, along with the spring onions, prawns and cucumbers.

5 Serve the salad garnished with lime wedges.

Curry ramen

for 2 servings

for 60 minutes

ingredients

30 grams of cashew nuts

30 grams of bacon, green

150 grams of ramen

200 grams of coconut milk

250 grams of ground pork

400 milliliters of chicken broth

½ - 1 teaspoon sambal oelek

1 tablespoon of katjap manis

1 tablespoon palm sugar, ground (alternatively brown sugar)

1 tablespoon of soy sauce

1-2 tablespoons of peanut oil

1-2 tablespoons sesame oil, light

2 tablespoons of curry paste, red

½ bunch of coriander greens

2-3 centimeters of ginger

1 organic lime; 1-2 shallots

2 eggs, size M

2 spring onions

2 cloves of garlic

sea-salt

preparation

1. Dice the bacon into ½ inch pieces. Peel and chop finely the garlic and ginger. Wash the spring onions, clean them thoroughly and cut the green and white parts into thin rings. Peel the shallots and cut them into fine rings. Rinse the coriander thoroughly, shake it dry, and chop roughly the leaves. Wash the lime under hot water, dry it with kitchen paper, and cut it into quarters.

2. Heat a wok and fry the cubes of bacon in it until translucent. Then add the cashews and the finely chopped shallots. Roast the whole thing over medium heat until everything turns a golden-brown color. Salt the contents of the wok then remove them with a slotted spoon and let them degrease on kitchen paper.

3. Put the sesame oil in a wok and turn the heat a little higher. Crumble in the ground beef and sear it, then let it cook for about 5 to 8 minutes until it is s crispy. Then stir in the ginger, ketjap manis, garlic, sambal oelek and soy sauce and taste the

minced meat. Pour the contents of the wok into a bowl and set it aside for now.

4 Poke the eggs and cook them in a small saucepan with boiling water for about 6 to 8 minutes until they are waxy. Chill the eggs under cold water and set them aside.

5 Put the peanut oil in the wok and toast it with the curry paste for a short moment. Deglaze the contents of the wok with the broth and coconut milk and let the contents of the wok simmer on low heat for about 6 to 8 minutes. Taste the sauce with the palm sugar.

6 Boil water in a large saucepan and cook the ramen in it. Peel the eggs and cut them in half.

7 Divide the ramen on bowls, pour the curry sauce over them, add the meat and serve the dish with the eggs and the quartered limes. To serve, sprinkle the whole thing with the cashew and bacon mixture, the spring onions and the coriander.

Dan Dan Ramen

for 4 servings

for 60 minutes

easily

ingredients

For the chili oil:

75 milliliters of oil

½ teaspoon of Chinese five-spice powder

1 tablespoon of sesame seeds

1 tablespoon of Sichuan peppercorns

2 tablespoons of pepper flakes, red

For the pork:

375 grams of ground pork

2 teaspoons of soy sauce

1 tablespoon of Chinese black vinegar

1 tablespoon of hoisin sauce

1 tablespoon of vegetable oil

For the sauce:

50 milliliters of tahini

1 tablespoon of Chinese black vinegar

1 tablespoon of honey

1 tablespoon of sesame oil, toasted

2 tablespoons of chili oil

2 tablespoons of ginger

2 tablespoons of soy sauce

3 tablespoons of water

3 cloves of garlic

For the garnish:

10 grams of coriander leaves

40 grams of roasted peanuts

500 grams of ramen

2 spring onions

preparation

1. Chop roughly the peanuts, put them in a pan and briefly toast them without fat. Wash the spring onions thoroughly then cut them into fine rings. Peel the ginger and garlic. Grate the ginger and finely chop the garlic.

2. Put the vegetable oil together with the Sichuan peppercorns in a small saucepan and heat both to 160 ° degrees. Then pull the pot off the stove and add the spice mixture, pepper flakes and sesame seeds. Let the oil cool completely.

3. For the pork, put the vegetable oil in a large pan and heat it over medium heat. Add the pork and use a wooden spoon to chop it up. Then cook the meat until the meat turns golden and crispy. Then add the vinegar, the hoisin sauce and the soy sauce and cook everything until the liquid has completely evaporated.

4. Put all the ingredients for the sauce in a bowl and whisk them together well.

5. Cook the ramen al dente, then drain and drain well. Then add them to the sauce in the bowl and mix everything together well.

6. Divide the ramen in bowls, spread the pork on top and garnish the dish with roasted peanuts, spring onion rings and the coriander. Drizzle with a little more chili oil to serve.

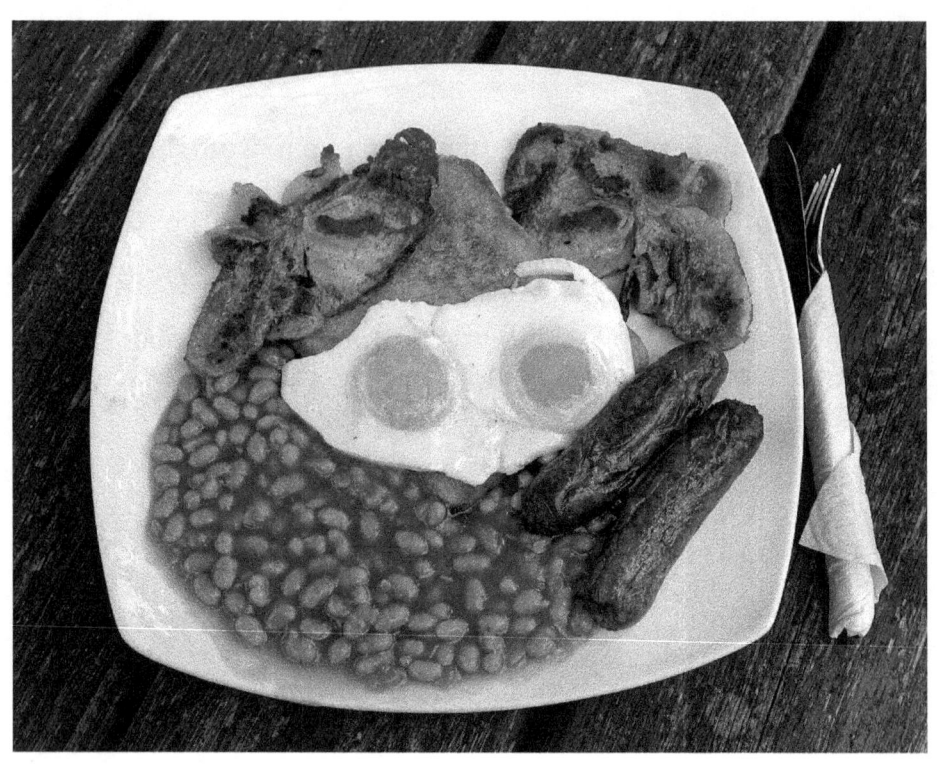

English Breakfast

for 2 servings

Less than30 minutes

easily

ingredients

100 grams of cheddar, grated

200 grams of ramen

1 teaspoon of extra virgin olive oil

3 slices of bacon

2 eggs, size M

2 spring onions

Sriracha

Pepper

preparation

1. Wash the spring onions thoroughly and cut them into fine rings. Chop the

bacon slices into pieces about 1 centimeter in size. Boil the ramen al dente, pour it off - catch 40 milliliters of the ramen water - and let it drain well. Then mix the ramen with the oil to avoid sticking together.

2   Heat a medium pan on medium heat and fry the pieces of bacon in it until they are crispy. Then add the ramen to the pan and coat them with the bacon fat and the bacon itself. Then pull the pan off the heat.

3   Using a fork, whisk the eggs in a bowl and stir in the grated cheese. Then add the mixture to the pan and mix it well with the ramen and bacon. Divide the dish in bowls and garnish with the spring onions, the pepper and the hot sauce as desired.

Peanut Curry Ramen

for 2 servings

less than 30 minutes

easily

ingredients

100 grams of peanut butter

250 grams of ramen

½ - 1 liter of dashi or vegetable stock

1 teaspoon curry paste, red

2 tablespoons of agave syrup

2 tablespoons of soy sauce

1 can of coconut milk (400 milliliters)

1 small piece of ginger

2 cloves of garlic

2 limes

10 shiitake mushrooms (alternatively mushrooms)

Chilies, peanuts, coriander, sesame seeds as desired

preparation

1 Heat a little oil in a pan. Clean the shiitake mushrooms, cut them into strips and fry them in the pan over high heat until they are significantly reduced.

2 Peel the ginger and garlic, chop both finely, reduce the pan to medium heat and fry the ginger and garlic together with the mushrooms for another 1 to 2 minutes.

3 Add 1 teaspoon of curry paste to the pan, fry it briefly and then remove the contents of the pan with the vegetable stock and coconut milk. At 500 milliliters this becomes a sauce - at 1 liter this dish becomes a soup. Then add the peanut butter and stir it in well.

4 When the peanut butter has dissolved, add 2 tablespoons of agave syrup, the juice of one lime and 2 tablespoons of soy sauce.

5 Add the ramen and let them cook. If necessary, add enough liquid to cover the ramen.

6 Remove the white core of the chili and then finely chop it. Chop the coriander, cut the lime into wedges then serve the pan with the chopped chili, coriander, and sesame seeds. Garnish the dish with cashews and peanuts to make it even more crispy.

Peanut ramen with sesame seeds

    for 4 servings

less than30 minutes

easily

ingredients

200 grams of edamame

375 grams of ramen

80 milliliters of soy sauce

200 milliliters of water

2 tablespoons of sesame oil

3 heaping tablespoons of peanut butter

3 level tablespoons of cornstarch

3 tablespoons of lemon juice

7 tablespoons of maple syrup

½ teaspoon pepper, ground

1 clove of garlic

2 carrots

some oil

some sesame

preparation

1 Mix the maple syrup with the peanut butter, sesame oil, soy sauce, cornstarch, water and lemon juice using a whisk to make a homogeneous sauce. Peel and chop the clove of garlic and add it to the sauce. Peel the carrots with a peeler and cut them into thin strips. Cook the ramen halfway then drain it off.

2 Put some oil in a pan, heat it up and fry the frozen edamame in it for about

2 minutes. Then add the sauce and let everything simmer over medium heat. Then add the carrot strips and the ramen and stir the whole thing again and again until the sauce is evenly distributed over the ramen. As soon as the sauce takes on a creamy consistency and is on all the ramen, the pan can be removed from the heat. Arrange the contents of the pan in bowls and sprinkle with a handful of sesame seeds to serve.

Refreshing Chicken Ramen

for 2 servings

for 60 minutes

ingredients

35 grams of tempura dough mix

40 grams of ginger, pickled

200 grams of chicken breast

400 grams of ramen

800 milliliters of chicken stock

2 tablespoons of mirin

2 tablespoons miso paste, light

4 tablespoons of sake

1 handful of baby spinach leaves

¼ cucumber

½ small carrot

preparation

1 Boil the stock in a large saucepan over high heat and then let it boil for about 15 minutes until the liquid is reduced to 400 milliliters. Then mix in the mirin, miso paste and sake and let everything cool down well. Meanwhile, peel the cucumber and carrot and cut them lengthways into strips using a Julienne cutter. Wash the spinach and shake it dry. Drain the ginger well and then cut it into fine strips.

2 Cook the ramen al dente, drain, rinse with cold water, and then drain well. Pat the chicken breast dry with a paper towel.

3 Mix the tempura batter mixture with 50 milliliters of water to a smooth consistency.

4 Fill the pan with about 1 centimeter high of oil and heat it to about 180 degrees. Then pull the chicken breast through the batter mixture and fry them in the hot oil for around 3 to 4 minutes on each side. Then cut the chicken breast into strips around 5 millimeters wide.

5 Spread the vegetables, ginger, stock and ramen in bowls. Using a fork, turn the ramen up in a spiral and serve the chicken in the bowl.

Prawn ramen

for 2 servings

less than 30 minutes

easily

ingredients

10 grams of bonito flakes

15 grams of kombu algae, dried

15 grams of mung bean sprouts (alternatively bean sprouts)

30 grams of baby spinach leaves

30 grams of sea lettuce algae

100 grams of shrimp, peeled, raw

400 grams of ramen

800 milliliters of fish stock

1 teaspoon of garlic oil

6 tablespoons of soy sauce

1 egg, size M

preparation

1. Boil the stock in a large saucepan and let it boil down on high heat for 10 minutes until it reduces to 600 milliliters. Then add the kombu seaweed, remove the pan from the stove and let it steep for about 13 minutes. Then add the bonito flakes and let everything stand for another 2 minutes. Then pour everything through a sieve, catching the stock and pouring it back into the pot. Remove the kombu seaweed and bonito flakes.

2. Rinse the mung bean sprouts thoroughly and let them drain well. Pick the spinach, wash it, and shake it dry. Heat water in a small saucepan and cook the egg in it for 6 minutes until it is waxy. Immediately remove the egg from the pot, rinse it with cold water, peel it and let it cool completely in ice water. Then cut the egg in half lengthways.

3. Reheat the stock. Then put the prawns in the hot, but not boiling stock and let everything stand for about 3 to 4 minutes until the prawns are cooked. Then take it out and set it aside.

4. Cook the ramen al dente and drain.

5. Distribute 3 tablespoons of the soy sauce in each of the bowls and pour the stock over them. Add the ramen and use a fork to twist them up in a spiral.

6. Arrange the egg, prawns, spinach, sprouts and wakame on top. Sprinkle the garlic oil on the ramen and serve immediately.

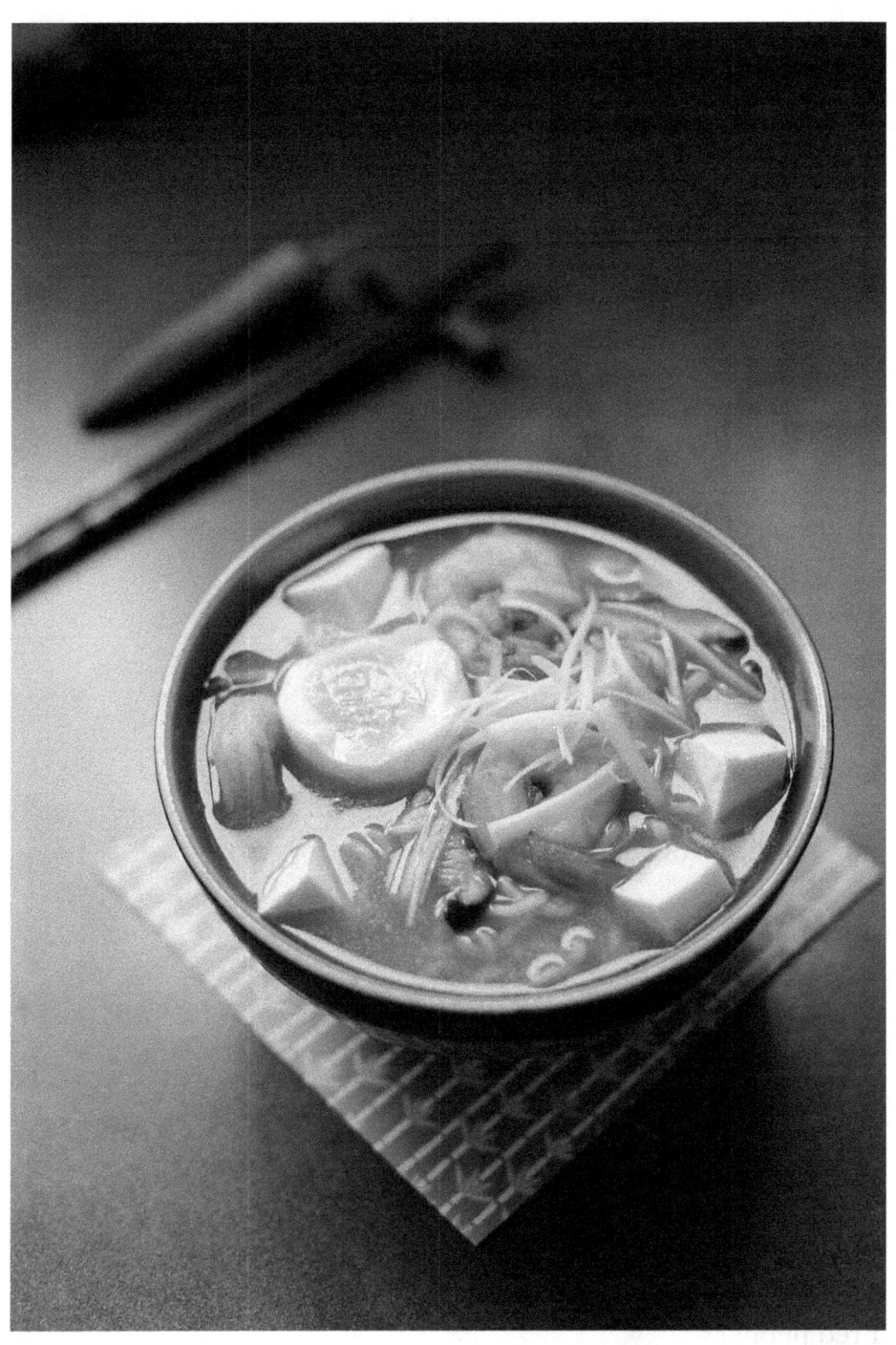

Shrimp Garlic Ramen

for 4 servings

for 30 minutes

easily

ingredients

45 grams of sugar, brown

300 grams of ramen

500 grams of shrimp

75 milliliters of soy sauce

150 milliliters of vegetable broth

1 teaspoon of ginger

2 teaspoons of sriracha

1 tablespoon of vegetable oil

1 tablespoon of sesame oil

1 large broccoli

1 red pepper

1 lime, the juice of it

2 spring onions

2 cloves of garlic

Black pepper

salt

preparation

1. Wash the broccoli thoroughly and divide it into florets. Wash the spring onions and cut them into thin slices. Peel the ginger and garlic, finely chop both. Wash and clean the peppers thoroughly and cut them into thin slices.

2. Cook the ramen al dente, then drain and drain well.

3. In a large pan, heat the vegetable oil over high heat. Add the prawns, season them with pepper and salt and cook them for about 2 minutes on each side until they become opaque. Remove the prawns from the pan and set them aside.

4. Then reduce the heat to low to medium, add the sesame oil to the pan and fry the ginger and garlic for 1 minute. Then deglaze both with the vegetable stock and stir in the lime juice, soy sauce, sriracha and brown sugar. Boil the whole thing, reduce the heat again and let everything simmer for about 5 minutes until the sauce thickens.

5. Add the broccoli and bell peppers to the pan and cover them and cook the vegetables for about 5 minutes until they are tender.

6 Put the shrimp back in the pan and stir everything together so that the shrimp are completely coated in the sauce.

7 Add the spring onions and ramen and stir well. Then divide the dish into bowls and serve garnished with the sriracha.

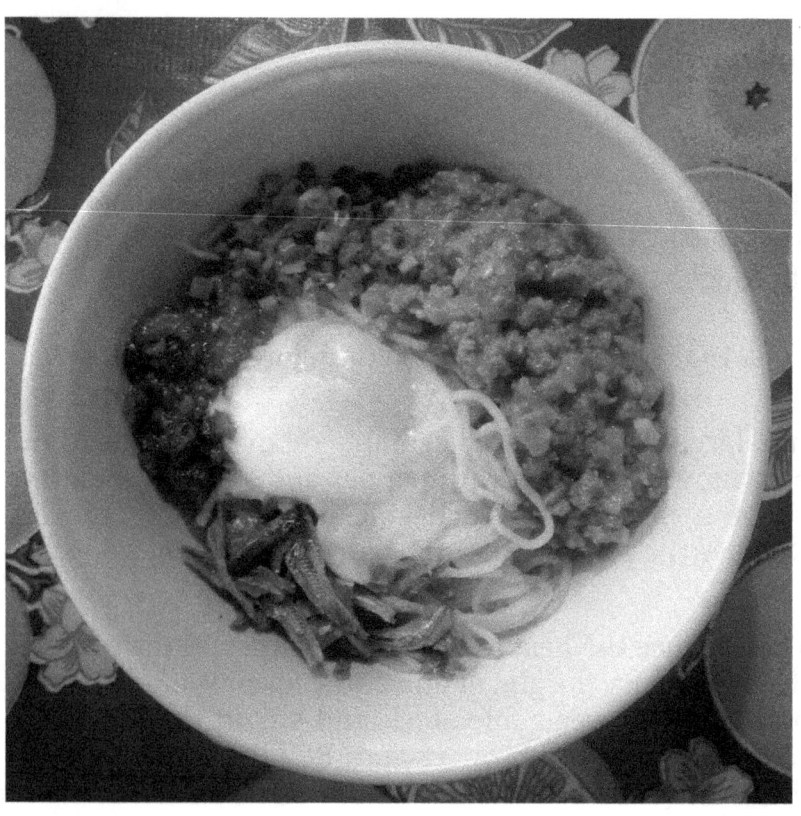

Fried ramen

    for 4 servings

for 30 minutes

easily

ingredients

For the ramen:

100 grams of shiitake mushrooms, sliced

150 grams of ramen

1 teaspoon ginger, grated

2 tablespoons of oil

½ bunch of coriander, chopped

1 broccoli, cut into florets

1 clove of garlic, chopped

3 carrots, cut into thin strips

pepper

salt

For the sauce:

1 teaspoon ginger, grated

2 teaspoons of sugar, brown

1 tablespoon of hoisin sauce

2 tablespoons rice vinegar

2 tablespoons of sesame oil

4 tablespoons of soy sauce

preparation

1 Put the ingredients for the sauce in a bowl and whisk them thoroughly.

2 Cook the ramen until soft, then drain and drain well.

3 Heat the oil in a wok and fry the vegetables in it for about 5 minutes on medium heat while stirring. Then season it with the ginger, pepper and salt.

4 Push the vegetables to the edge of the wok and place the ramen in the middle. Pour the sauce over it and mix everything together thoroughly. Continue frying the dish for 2 minutes.

5 Divide everything into bowls and fold in the coriander just before serving.

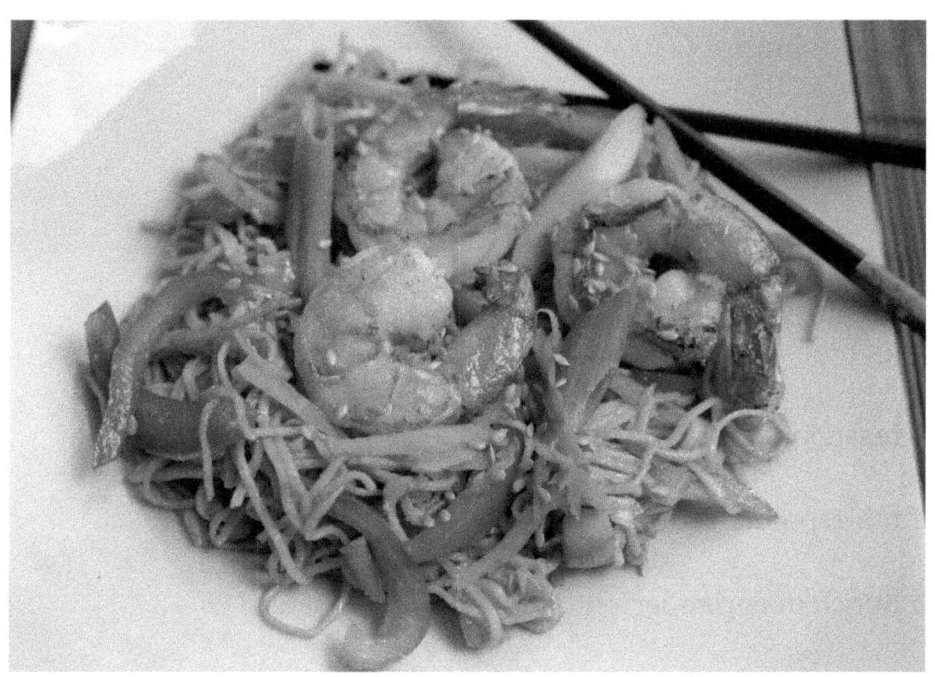

Grilled chicken ramen

for 3 servings

for 30 minutes

ingredients

300 grams of ramen

1.25 liters of chicken broth

1 teaspoon of neutral oil

1 tablespoon of soy sauce

1 bunch of coriander

2 handfuls of kale

1 thumb-sized piece of ginger

½ onion, red; 1 chili

1 clove of garlic

1 lime, the juice of it

1 Pak Choi

2 skinless chicken breast fillets

preparation

1. Wash, core and slice the chili. Peel the ginger, garlic and onion, chop the ginger and cut the garlic and onion into thin slices. Wash the cilantro, shake it dry, and finely chop it. Wash and clean the pak choi and quarter it lengthways.

2. Put the chili, the chicken stock, the ginger, the garlic and the soy sauce in a large pan and bring everything to a boil. Cover and let the pan simmer for about 15 minutes.

3. Meanwhile, place the meat between two pieces of cling film and use a rolling pin to pound it about 1 centimeter thick. Season the meat well and drizzle with oil.

4. Heat a pan on medium to high heat and cook the chicken in it for about 4 to 5 minutes per side. Then let the chicken rest on a plate for 5 minutes, covered with cling film, and then cut it into slices.

5. Add the pak choi and ramen to the broth and simmer for 2 minutes before adding the kale and simmering for 1 more minute.

6. Spread the soup with the filler in bowls, pour the broth over them, spread the chicken and garnish the dish with the chilies, ginger, coriander, lime juice and onions.

Vegetable ramen

for 2 servings

for 30 minutes

ingredients

For the ramen:

400 grams of ramen

1 tablespoon of sesame seeds, toasted

2 tablespoons of peanut oil

1 handful of mushrooms, brown, quartered

1 thumb-sized piece of ginger, finely diced

1 small broccoli, cut into florets

1 chili, diced

1 carrot, thinly sliced

2 spring onions, cut into thin rings

2 cloves of garlic, sliced

For the sauce:

1 teaspoon sesame oil

2-3 teaspoons of powdered sugar

1 tablespoon of chili oil

3 tablespoons of Chinese vinegar, black

5 tablespoons soy sauce, light

preparation

1   Put the ingredients for the sauce in a bowl and stir them together thoroughly.

2   Boil the broccoli florets in boiling water for about 1 minute, then drain, shred, and set aside.

3   Heat the wok, heat 1 tablespoon of peanut oil in it and stir-fry the carrot for

1 minute. Then add the chili and garlic and fry both for 1 more minute while stirring. Add the broccoli, mushrooms, and ginger and cook for 2 minutes.

4   Add the ramen to the pot and stir-fry for 1 minute. Deglaze the whole thing

with the sauce and briefly boil it until the sugar starts to caramelize. Then, pull the wok off the stove and let the contents steep for 1 minute.

5 Spread the dish in bowls and serve garnished with the spring onions and sesame seeds.

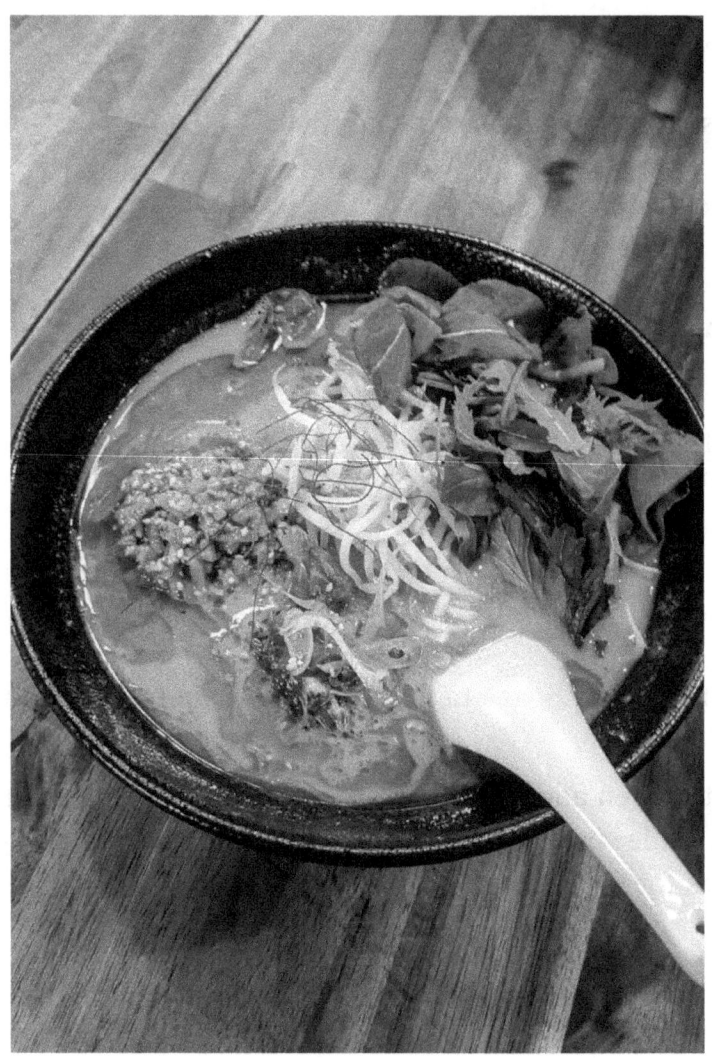

Vegetable beef ramen

for 4 servings

less than 30 minutes

easily

ingredients

100 grams of mung bean sprouts

240 grams of ramen

400 grams of carrots, thinly sliced

500 grams of beef minute steaks, thinly sliced

600 milliliters of meat bouillon

½ teaspoon of salt

2 tablespoons of peanut oil

2 tablespoons of coriander

2 tablespoons soy sauce, light

6 spring onions, thinly sliced

pepper

preparation

1 Heat some oil in a pan and fry the meat in portions for 1 minute each while stirring. Season the meat and remove it from the pan.

2 Fry the carrots in the roasting set for about 5 minutes then add the spring onions. Fry the whole thing for another 2 minutes and remove both from the pan.

3 Pour the stock and soy sauce into the pan, bring to the boil then reduce the heat.

4 Cook the ramen al dente, then drain and drain well. Then place them in bowls, place the meat, vegetables, and mung bean sprouts on top, and sprinkle with coriander to serve.

All sorts of green

for 2 servings

less than 30 minutes

easily

ingredients

10 grams of shiitake mushrooms, dried

15 grams of kombu algae, dried

60 grams of edamame beans, peeled, frozen

60 grams of vegetables, pickled sweet and sour

60 grams of pointed cabbage

100 grams of romanesco

400 grams of ramen

800 milliliters vegetable stock

1 tablespoon of rapeseed oil

2 tablespoons of sesame dressing, toasted salt

preparation

1. Thaw the edamame, rinse it, and let it drain well. Meanwhile, divide the Romanesco into florets and then halve or quarter them. Wash the cabbage thoroughly and cut it into strips.

2. Boil the stock and then add the kombu algae and the shiitake mushrooms. Cover and let stand for 2 minutes and then remove the kombu algae. Let the contents of the pot stand for another 8 minutes and then remove the shiitake mushrooms. Then let the stock boil open again for 5 minutes until it has reduced to 600 milliliters. Discard the mushrooms.

3. Heat the oil in a pan and sear both the edamame and the romanesco for about 6 to 7 minutes. Then cook the ramen al dente, drain and drain well.

4. Distribute 1 tablespoon of the sesame dressing and ½ teaspoon of salt on each of the bowls and pour the contents of the bowl over the hot stock. Then add the ramen and use a fork to twist them up in a spiral.

5. Pour off the sweet and sour vegetables and serve them together with the edamame, romanesco and pointed cabbage on the ramen. Serve immediately.

Guacamole bowl

for 2 servings

for 30 minutes

ingredients

For the guacamole:

1 avocado, peeled, diced

100 milliliters of coconut milk, shaken well ½ teaspoon of salt

1 teaspoon jalapeño, chopped

1 teaspoon garlic, chopped

1 heaped tablespoon of coriander leaves, roughly chopped

½ lime, the juice from it

½ lemon, the juice from it

1 shallot, roughly chopped

For the prawns:

500 grams of shrimp, peeled, deveined, washed

½ teaspoon of allspice

1 teaspoon creole spice

1 teaspoon of olive oil

1 tablespoon of olive oil

1 pinch of salt

½ lime, the juice from it

For the bowl:

160 grams of cherry tomatoes, halved

300 grams of ramen

1 tablespoon of dill leaves, chopped

1 tablespoon coriander leaves, chopped

1 small cucumber, sliced

cooked pieces of bacon

preparation

1. Put all the ingredients for the guacamole in a blender and puree them to a homogeneous mass. You can adjust the consistency by using more lime or lemon juice or water. Season the guacamole with salt and set aside.

2. Prepare the shrimp. To do this, put 1 tablespoon of oil in a large pan and

heat it over medium heat until the oil begins to shimmer. Add the prawns to the pan with 1 teaspoon of olive oil and the remaining marinade ingredients and cook the prawns for a while. Then turn them once and cook them until they become opaque. Remove the pan from the stove and set the shrimp aside.

3. Cook the ramen al dente, then drain and drain well. Then place the ramen in a large bowl and add about ¾ of the guacamole, dill and a large pinch of coriander. Gently mix the herbs, ramen, and sauce together. Then add the cucumbers and tomatoes, fold them in and garnish the salad with the prawns, the remaining guacamole, the herbs and the pieces of bacon.

Ramen with meatballs

    for 4 servings

for 30 minutes

easily

ingredients

45 grams of sugar, brown

80 grams of breadcrumbs

300 grams of ramen

500 grams of minced meat

75 milliliters of soy sauce

110 milliliters of chicken broth

2 teaspoons of ginger

2 teaspoons of sesame oil

2 tablespoons of hoisin sauce

1 egg; 2 cloves of garlic

3 spring onions

Red pepper flakes

Black pepper

Vegetable oil

salt

sesame

preparation

1   Wash the spring onions thoroughly and cut them into fine rings. Peel the ginger and garlic and finely chop them.

2   Put the minced meat in a bowl along with the egg, half of the spring onions, garlic, breadcrumbs and 1 teaspoon of sesame oil. Season the whole thing with the paprika flakes, pepper and salt and knead the mixture well together. Use a tablespoon to form meatballs out of the mixture and roll them into balls.

3   Heat some oil in a pan over medium to high heat and fry the meatballs for about 2 minutes on each side until a crust is formed. Then remove the balls from the pan and add the remaining sesame oil.

4   Stir in the ginger and fry it for about 30 seconds. Then deglaze the contents of the pan with the chicken stock and stir in the hoisin sauce, soy sauce, and brown sugar. Cook the whole thing and add the meatballs back in. Then cover and let the pan simmer for about 10 more minutes.

5   Meanwhile, cook the ramen al dente, pour them off and let them drain well.

6 Put the ramen in the pan and stir in until the sauce is coated. Then divide

the pan's contents into bowls and garnish the dish with the remaining spring onions and the sesame seeds.

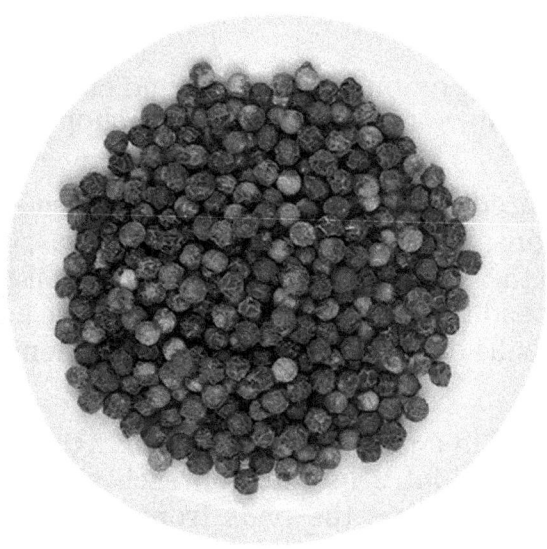

Chicken ramen with lime

for 2 servings

for 30 minutes

ingredients

60 grams of bamboo shoots, pickled

200 grams of chicken breast

300 grams of mini pak choi

400 grams of ramen

800 milliliters of chicken stock

1 tablespoon of rapeseed oil

4 tablespoons of sake

6 tablespoons of soy sauce

1 organic lime

1 spring onion

preparation

1. Boil the stock in a wide saucepan and let it simmer on high heat for around

10 minutes until it has reduced to 600 milliliters. In the meantime, wash and clean the spring onions and cut them into fine rings. Wash and clean the pak choi as well, then cut it into pieces of about two centimeters. Wash the lime thoroughly with hot water then dry it with a paper towel. Use a zest peeler to peel off the peel of the lime. Rinse the sprouts and let them drain well.

2 Pat the chicken breast dry with a paper towel. Heat some oil in a pan over medium heat and fry the meat in it for about 4 to 5 minutes on each side. Glaze the meat with 1 tablespoon of soy sauce, then cut it into strips about 5 millimeters thick.

3 Cook the ramen al dente, then drain and drain well. Mix the rest of the soy sauce with the sake and divide the whole thing into bowls. Pour the hot stock on top of the liquid, add the ramen and use a fork to turn them up in a spiral.

4 Finally, arrange the spring onions, the chicken, the lime zest, the pak choi and the sprouts on the dish.

Hoisin ramen

for 4 servings

less than 30 minutes

easily

ingredients

150 grams of ramen

500 grams of pork tenderloin

40 milliliters of water

50 milliliters of hoisin sauce

2 tablespoons of butter

3 tablespoons of soy sauce

3 tablespoons of sugar

3 cloves of garlic

spring onions

Pepper flakes, red

preparation

1   Wash the spring onions and cut them into fine slices. Peel the garlic and chop finely it. Crush the pepper flakes.

2   Preheat the oven to 240 degrees.

3   Put the hoisin sauce, garlic, pepper flakes, soy sauce and sugar in a saucepan and mix them together.

4   Line a baking sheet with parchment paper. Grease a wire rack and place it on the baking sheet. Place the fillet on the grid and brush it with 40 milliliters of the sauce mixture. Put the whole thing in the preheated oven for about 15 to 20 minutes until the internal temperature of the fillet reaches 145 degrees.

5   Mix the rest of the sauce mixture with the water and boil it in a small saucepan. Then reduce the heat and simmer the sauce for about 5 minutes, stirring occasionally. Remove the saucepan from the stove and stir in the butter.

6   Take the meat out of the oven and let it rest for 5 minutes. Then cut it into slices. Meanwhile, cook the ramen al dente, drain and drain well.

7   Divide the ramen in bowls, add the meat and spring onions, and pour the sauce over them.

Ginger Chicken Ramen

for 2 servings

for 60 minutes

ingredients

20 grams of ginger, red, pickled

60 grams of sea lettuce algae

200 grams of chicken breast

400 grams of ramen

800 milliliters of chicken stock

2 tablespoons miso paste, light

2 tablespoons of rapeseed oil

1 egg, size M

1 spring onion

1 clove of garlic

preparation

1   Wash and clean the spring onions, then cut them into fine rings. Peel the garlic and chop finely it.

2   Heat water in a small saucepan and cook the egg in it for about 6 minutes until it is soft as wax. Immediately remove the egg from the pot, rinse it with cold water, peel it and let it cool completely in ice water. Then cut the egg in half lengthways. Peel the ginger and cut it into sticks.

3   Boil the stock in a large saucepan and heat it for 10 minutes on high heat until it has reduced to 600 milliliters.

4   Meanwhile, pat the chicken breast dry with a paper towel. Heat 1 tablespoon of oil in a pan and sear the meat on both sides on medium heat for around 4 to 5 minutes each time. Turn off the stove, add the garlic and the rest of the oil and fry both for a short moment. Then cut the chicken diagonally into thin slices 3 millimeters thick.

5   Cook the ramen al dente, drain and drain well. Spread the miso paste on bowls and pour the hot stock over them. Add the ramen and use a fork to twist them up in a spiral. Then serve the egg, spring onions, chicken, ginger, and wakame on top.

6   Drizzle the garlic oil that is left in the pan on the ramen and serve the dish straight away.

Ginger beef ramen

for 4 servings

less than 30 minutes

easily

ingredients

125 grams of green beans

200 grams of ramen

500 grams of flank steak

120 milliliters soy sauce

1 teaspoon red chili flakes

1 tablespoon rice vinegar

5 centimeters of ginger

1 large carrot

1 clove of garlic

preparation

1   Mash the chili flakes with a spoon. Wash the beans thoroughly and chop them up. Peel the ginger and garlic and finely chop them. Wash the carrot thoroughly and cut it into thin slices. Put the chili flakes along with the ginger, garlic, rice vinegar and soy sauce in a medium-sized bowl and mix everything together well.

2   Heat some oil in a large pan over medium to high heat. Then add the steak and cook for 3 minutes on each side. Then place the steak on a cutting board to rest. Put the beans, carrots, and sauce in the pan together and mix everything together well. Let it simmer for about 5 minutes.

3   Meanwhile, cut the steak into slices and then add it to the pan with the ramen. Mix everything together well, divide it into bowls and serve.

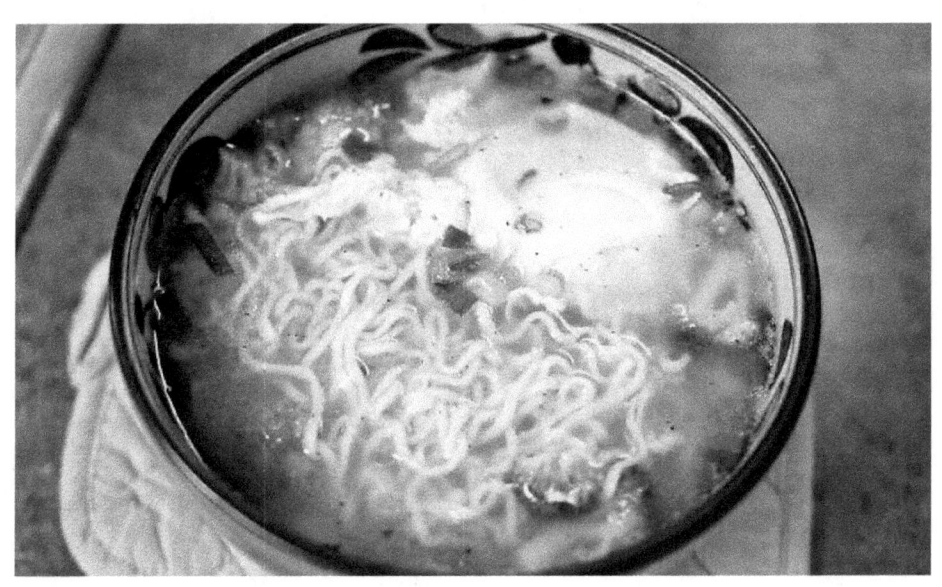

Ginger-lemongrass ramen

for 2 servings

for 30 minutes

ingredients

100 grams of ramen

1 handful of baby spinach leaves

5 slices of ginger

1 chili, red

1 chicken breast fillet

1 clove of garlic

1 lemongrass

Lemon wedges

preparation

1   Boil 300 milliliters of water in a pan. Wash the chili thoroughly and cut it in half. Leave one half of the chili whole and finely chop the other half. Chop the chicken breast into small pieces. Peel and chop the garlic. Wash the spinach, shake it dry, and mince it.

2 Add the whole half of the chili, the ginger, the garlic and the lemongrass and stir in well. Let the pan simmer for about 5 minutes and then remove the solid ingredients. Instead, add the ramen and cook for about 2 minutes.

3 Add the spinach and chicken breast to the pan to warm up.

4 Divide the dish in bowls and garnish with the chopped chili and lemon wedges.

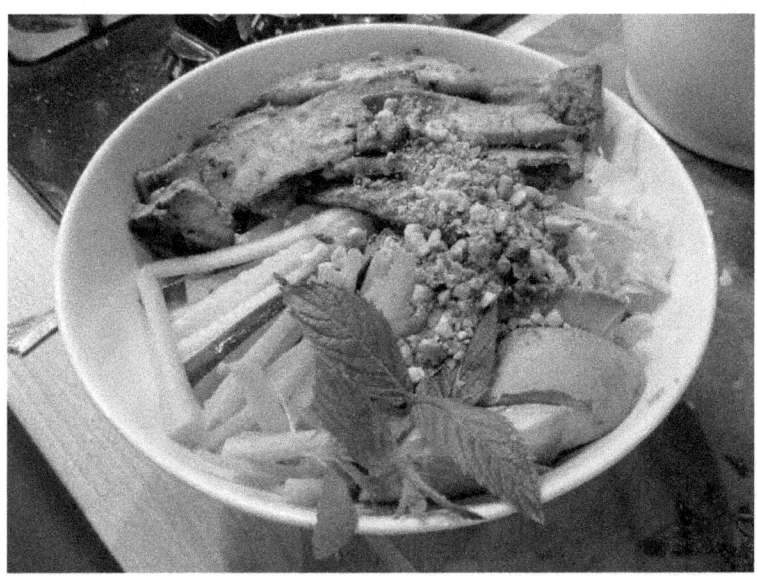

Scallop and asparagus ramen

    for 4 servings

less than 30 minutes

easily

ingredients

100 grams of chicken

500 grams of scallops

500 grams of asparagus

1 teaspoon paprika sauce

1 teaspoon sesame oil

1 tablespoon of lime juice

1 tablespoon of olive oil

2 tablespoons of soy sauce

1 clove of garlic

1 red pepper

3 spring onions

preparation

1   Halve the scallops horizontally. Wash the spring onions thoroughly and cut them thinly. Peel and chop the garlic. Wash the peppers and cut them into thin slices using a peeler. Peel and clean the asparagus, then cut it into 2 ½ centimeters long pieces.

2   Cook the ramen al dente, then drain and drain well.

3   Heat some oil in a large pan and briefly fry the peppers and asparagus in it until they are crispy. Add the spring onions and garlic and cook for 1 minute. Stir in the scallops and fry them until they turn opaque.

4   Mix in the lime juice, paprika sauce, sesame oil and soy sauce and mix the contents of the pan together well.

5   Divide the ramen in bowls and distribute the pan's contents on top.

Cheese ramen

for 3 servings

less than 30 minutes

easily

ingredients

150 grams of ramen

180 grams of cheese mix

300 milliliters of milk, low in fat

2 teaspoons of flour

2 tablespoons of butter, salted

Cherry tomatoes, halved

Parsley, chopped

preparation

1 Cook the ramen al dente, then drain and drain well.

2 Melt butter in a saucepan and stir in the flour, cook while stirring for 30 seconds. Then add the milk and cheese and cook

the whole thing while stirring on medium speed until the cheese has melted.

3   Add the ramen to the pot and stir well. Then pull the pot off the stove and let everything steep for about 2 to 3 minutes.

4   Divide the dish in bowls and garnish with the cherry tomatoes and parsley.

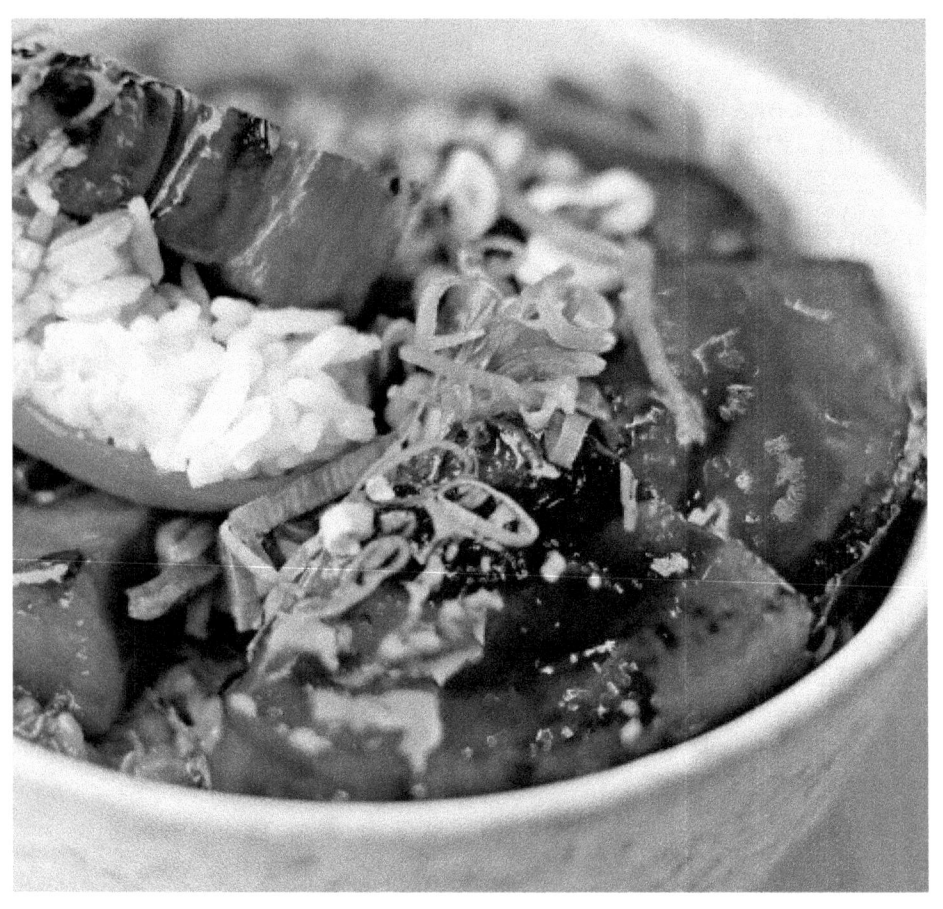

Garlic ramen

for 2 servings

less than 30 minutes

easily

ingredients

100 grams of ramen

225 milliliters of chicken broth

¼ teaspoon salt

1 teaspoon parsley, dried

3 tablespoons unsalted butter

3 large cloves of garlic

2 pinches of black pepper

preparation

1 Peel and chop the garlic cloves. Then place the chopped garlic cloves in a medium pan along with 2 tablespoons of the butter. Cook the pan's contents over medium heat, stirring constantly, until the garlic turns a light golden color.

2   Then add the chicken broth, pepper and salt and cook them as well. Add the ramen and cook, stirring, for 20 to 30 seconds.

3   Cook the contents of the pan until most of the liquid has evaporated and only a little of the broth is left. Then, pull the pan off the stove and stir in the remaining butter and dried parsley.

4   Put the ramen in bowls and serve directly.

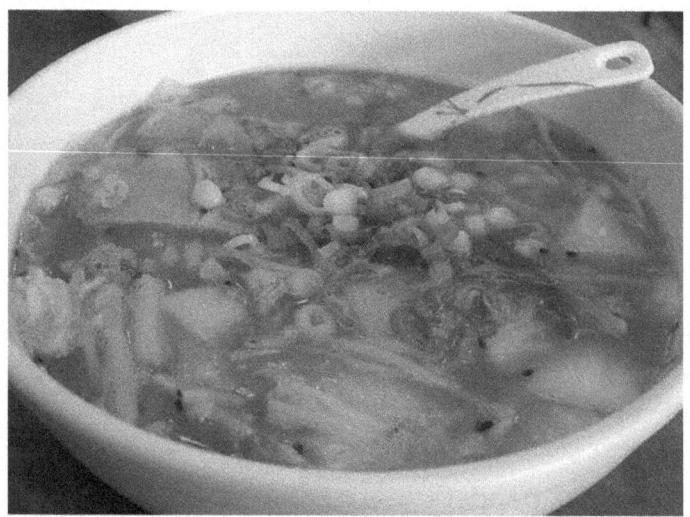

Garlic Sesame Ramen

for 4 servings less than 30 minutes easily

ingredients

100 grams of ramen

40 milliliters soy sauce

1 teaspoon sugar, brown

2 teaspoons of sesame oil

2 teaspoons of sriracha

2 cloves of garlic

spring onions

preparation

1   Cook the ramen al dente, then drain and drain well.

2   Heat the sesame oil in a pan or saucepan over medium heat. Peel and chop the garlic, then sauté for 2 minutes, stirring constantly.

3   Whisk the garlic in the pot with the soy sauce, sriracha and brown sugar until a homogeneous liquid forms. Then add the ramen and let them heat up for a short time.

4 Wash the spring onions and cut them into fine rings. Put the ramen in bowls and garnish with the spring onions.

Coconut ramen

for 4 servings

for 120 minutes

easy

ingredients

For the ramen:

50 grams of beans, halved

50 grams of bean sprouts

80 grams of ramen

100 grams of shrimp, peeled, deveined

100 grams of carrots, cut into sticks

125 milliliters of coconut milk

500 milliliters of beef soup

2 tablespoons of chili oil

2 tablespoons of olive oil

1 pak choi, halved lengthways, cut crosswise into strips

2 cloves of garlic, finely chopped

4 spring onions, cut into 1cm wide pieces

pepper

salt

For the sauce:

20 grams of ginger, cut into small pieces

100 grams of onions, cut into small pieces

125 milliliters of red wine

250 milliliters soy sauce, sweet

3 teaspoons paprika powder, noble sweet

1 chili, cut into small pieces

2 cloves of garlic, cut into small pieces

preparation

1. Mix the paprika powder with the soy sauce and the wine, then stir in the

chili, ginger, garlic and onions and let everything simmer for about 1 hour on low heat. Then puree the chili sauce with the hand blender.

2   Heat some oil in a wok and fry the prawns in it. Add the vegetables and

garlic and fry everything. Deglaze the whole thing with the soup and stir in the chili sauce and coconut milk. Let the wok contents simmer for 5 minutes then season them with salt and pepper.

3   Spread the whole thing in bowls and pour the soup over it.

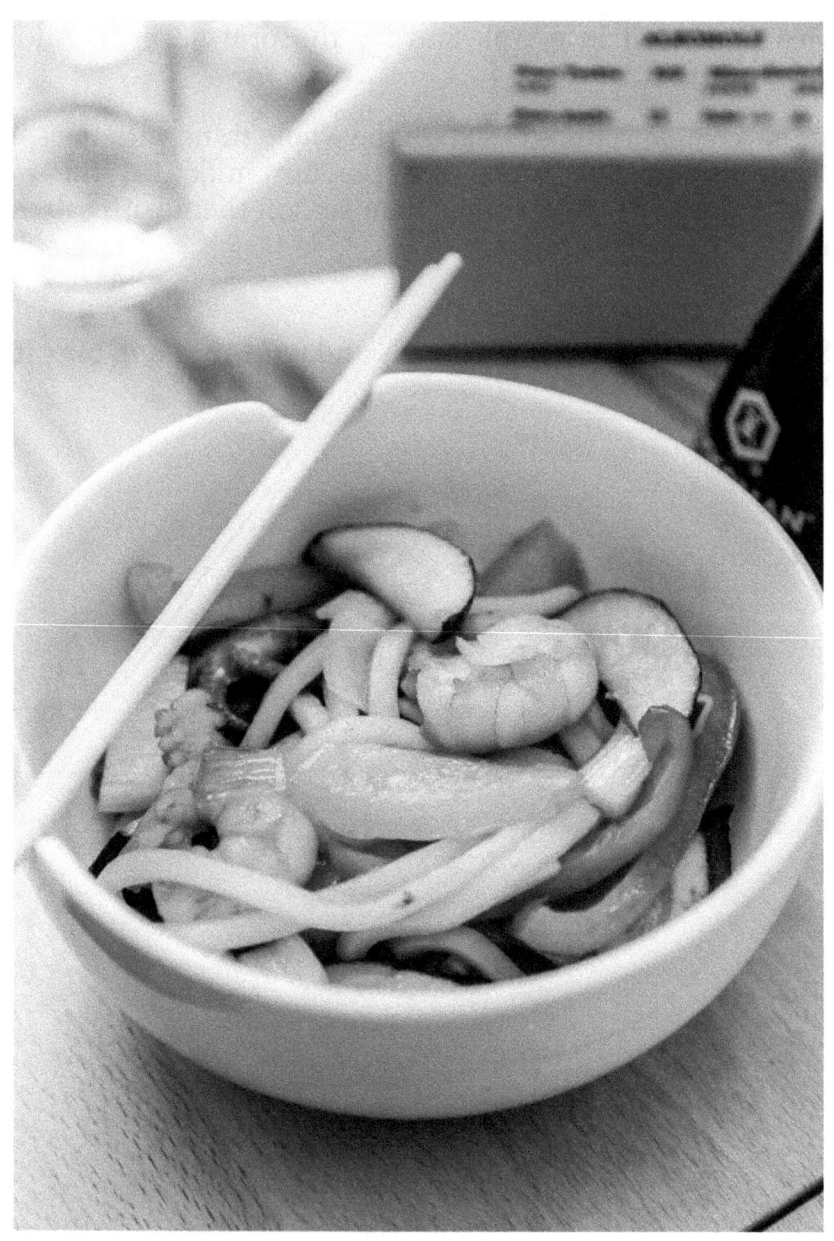

Salmon ramen

for 2 servings

for 60 minutes

ingredients

40 grams of ginger, pickled

100 grams of shrimp, peeled, raw

100 grams of smoked salmon

400 grams of ramen

800 milliliters of fish stock

½ teaspoon wasabi paste

6 tablespoons of soy sauce

1 spring onion

1 small pak choi

4 nori sheets, toasted salt

preparation

1   Pat the prawns dry with kitchen paper and cut them into fine cubes. Form six walnut-sized balls on it.

2 Cut the salmon into strips about 1 centimeter wide. Wash and clean the

spring onions, then cut them into fine rings. Drain the ginger well and wash and clean the pak choi in the meantime. Quarter the pak choi lengthways and then blanch it in boiling salted water for about 2 minutes. Then frighten off the pak choi and let it drain well.

3 Boil the stock in a wide saucepan and then let it cook on high heat for

around 10 minutes until it has reduced to 600 milliliters. Reduce the heat a little and wait until the stock stops boiling. Then add the shrimp balls and let them cook for about 3 minutes.

4 Spread the soy sauce and ¼ teaspoon of wasabi paste on the bowls and stir

both well together so that the paste dissolves. Then cook the ramen al dente, drain and drain well.

5 Remove the shrimp balls from the stock and pour them into the bowls. Add the ramen and use a fork to twist them up in a spiral.

6 Place the spring onions, shrimp balls, ginger, salmon and pak choi in the bowls and garnish the dish with the nori leaves on the edge of the bowl.

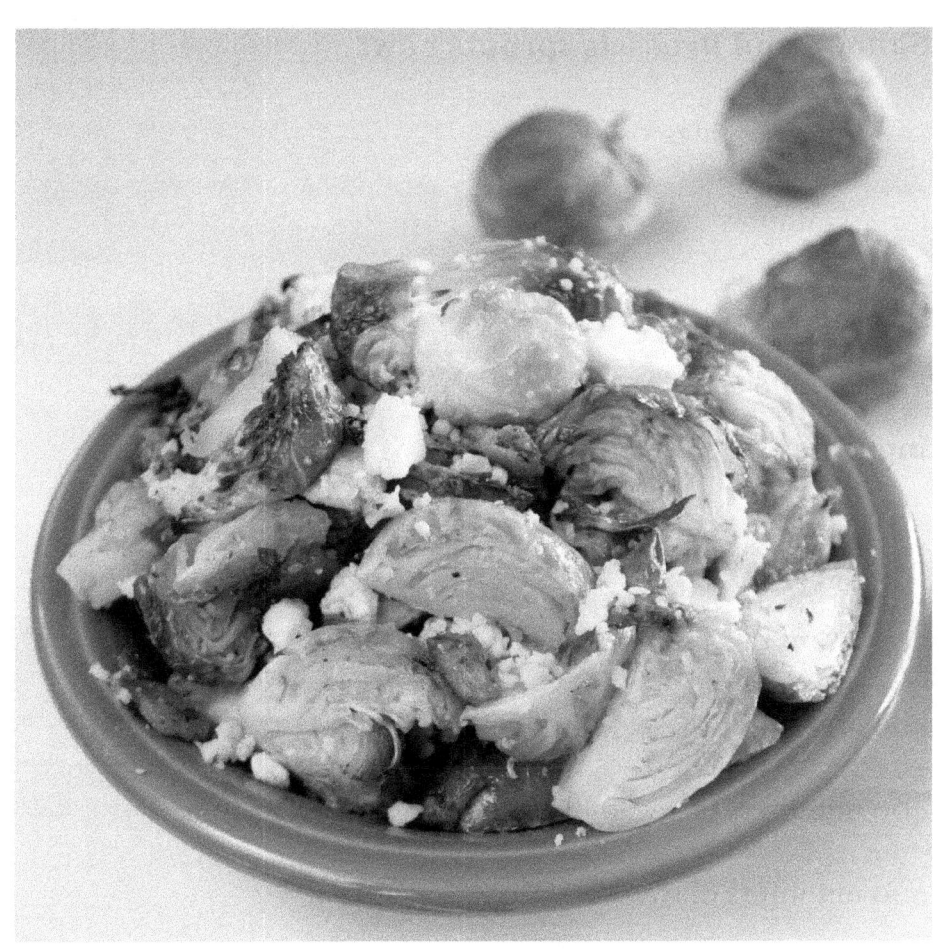

Salmon and Brussels sprouts bowl

for 2 servings

for 40 minutes

easily

ingredients

150 grams of ramen

200 grams of salmon

300 grams of Brussels sprouts

400 milliliters of vegetable stock

400 milliliters of water

1 teaspoon rapeseed oil

2 teaspoons of sesame seeds

3 teaspoons of Sambal Oelek

1 tablespoon of sesame oil

2 tablespoons of curry paste, red

2 tablespoons of miso paste

3 tablespoons of fish sauce

3 tablespoons of soy sauce

2 centimeters of ginger, chopped

1 spring onion, cut into rings

1 onion, chopped

2 eggs

2 cloves of garlic, chopped

preparation

1   Preheat the oven to 160 degrees.

2   Clean the Brussels sprouts, spread them on a baking sheet and then brush them with the sambal oelek. Cook the Brussels sprouts in the preheated oven for 20 minutes.

3   Meanwhile, heat the sesame oil in a large saucepan and briefly fry the

ginger, garlic and onion in it. Then deglaze the whole thing with the soy sauce, add the water, reduce the heat, and then let everything simmer for about 15 minutes.

4 Then strain the broth through a fine-mesh sieve into a saucepan and briefly

boil it. Reduce the heat and stir in the curry paste, vegetable stock, and miso paste. Add the ramen to the broth and let everything simmer for 7 minutes.

5 Put the eggs in a saucepan with boiling water and cook them until they are

waxy for about 6 minutes. Then shock them with cold water. Then peel them and cut them in half lengthways.

6 Heat the rapeseed oil in a pan and add the salmon. Then fry it on both sides for 3 minutes each and then deglaze it with the fish sauce.

7 Warm the Brussels sprouts in the broth and then divide the whole thing

into bowls. To serve, garnish with the spring onions, sprinkle the fish with the sesame seeds and then serve with the halved eggs.

Corn miso ramen

for 2 servings

for 60 minutes

ingredients

For the corn broth:

200 milliliters of soy milk

1 teaspoon vinegar

4 teaspoons of sesame oil

5 teaspoons of miso paste

5 teaspoons of soy sauce

2 tablespoons of tahini

3 centimeters of ginger

1 corn on the cob, fresh or pre-cooked

2 spring onions

4 cloves of garlic

4 shiitake mushrooms, dried

Also:

50 grams of soy fillets

150 grams of green leafy vegetables (kohlrabi leaves, Swiss chard, spinach, etc.)

250 grams of ramen

1 teaspoon sesame seeds

1 teaspoon sesame oil

2 teaspoons of soy sauce

preparation

1   Scald the shittake mushrooms and soy fillets with hot water and let them soak for about 20 minutes.

2   Meanwhile, wash the spring onions and cut their greens into fine rings, some of the white part into strips, and the rest into rings and place in cold water. Peel the ginger and garlic and finely chop them. Quarter the cob.

3   Heat the sesame oil in a saucepan and sauté the spring onion rings, ginger and garlic for 1 minute on a low heat. Add the miso paste and stir-fry for 2 minutes.

4   Add the vinegar, corn, shiitake mushrooms, soy milk, soy sauce, tahini and 800 milliliters of water, boil the whole thing and let it simmer for around 15 minutes on medium heat.

5   Boil the ramen until al dente, pour it off, frighten it off and let it drain well.

6 Marinate the soy fillets with 1 teaspoon of sesame oil and 1 teaspoon of soy sauce. Blanch the leafy vegetables in hot water for about 1 minute, then season them with 1 teaspoon of sesame seeds and 1 teaspoon of soy sauce.

7 Divide the ramen in bowls and pour the hot broth over them. Drape the toppings on top and serve the dish immediately.

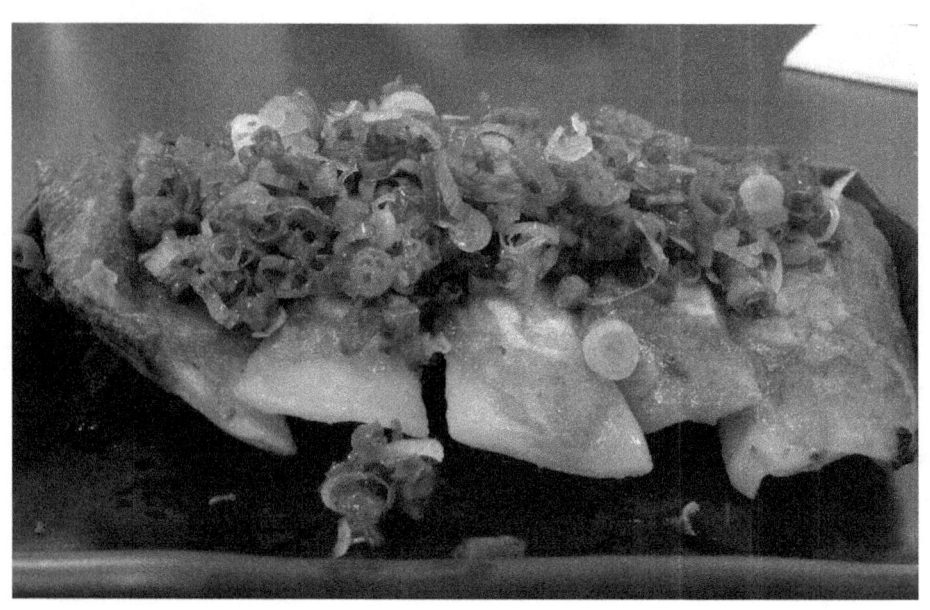

Matcha ramen (vegan)

for 2 servings

for 60 minutes

ingredients

20 grams of dried shiitake mushrooms

60 grams of bamboo shoots, pickled

60 grams of radish, yellow, pickled

100 grams of smoked tofu

400 grams of ramen

200 milliliters soy drink

800 milliliters vegetable stock

1 tablespoon of rapeseed oil

1 teaspoon matcha powder

2 tablespoons miso paste, light

2 tablespoons of nori flakes

preparation

1   Rinse the sprouts thoroughly and let them drain well. Let the radish drain well, then cut into fine slices and then into fine strips. Cut the tofu into slices around 5 millimeters thick then cut it into strips of the same thickness. Heat oil in a pan and fry the tofu in it for about 5 minutes until it becomes crispy.

2   Boil the stock together with the shiitake mushrooms in a large saucepan on high heat for about 10 minutes, reducing it to around 600 milliliters. Remove the shiitake mushrooms from the stock, then add the soy drink and reheat the stock - but make sure it doesn't boil again. Then cook the ramen al dente, drain and drain well.

3   Spread 1 tablespoon of the miso paste in each bowl. Then stir the matcha powder into the stock and also distribute it on the bowls. Then add the ramen and use a fork to twist them up in a spiral.

4   Serve the dish together with the radish, the sprouts and the tofu and finally sprinkle the ramen with the nori flakes.

Seafood ramen

for 2 servings

less than 30 minutes

easily

ingredients

200 grams of ramen

500 grams of seafood, mixed, frozen

2 tablespoons of oil

4 tablespoons sesame seeds, light

8 tablespoons of soy sauce

1 red pepper

preparation

1 Cook the ramen al dente, then drain and drain well. Thaw the seafood.

2 Heat 2 tablespoons of olive oil in a pan. Wash, core, and cut the peppers into strips. Then fry the pepper strips in the pan for 5 minutes.

3 Add the seafood, ramen, sesame seeds and soy sauce to the pan, stir everything together thoroughly, divide the dish into bowls and serve immediately.

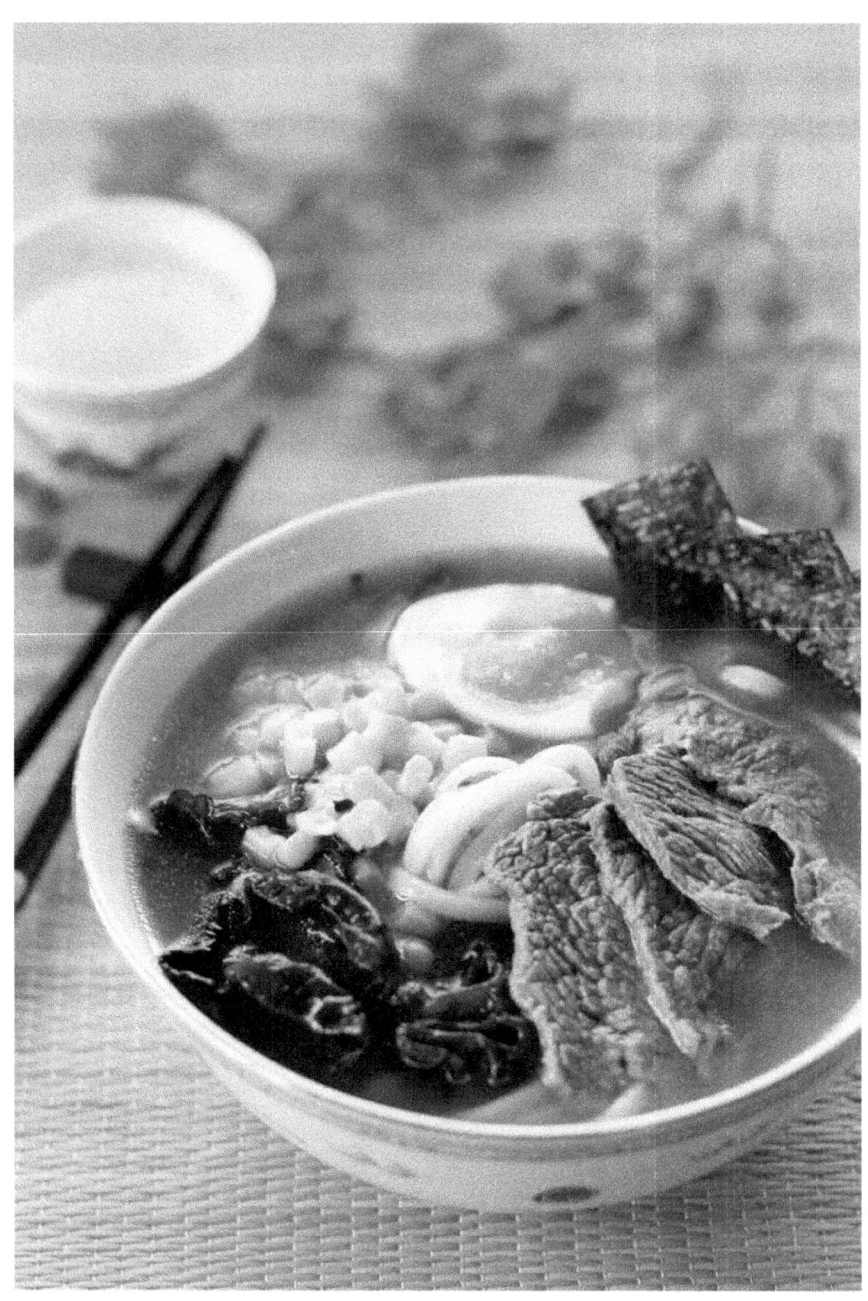

Minute ramen

for 4 servings

less than30 minutes

easily

ingredients

20 grams of coconut fat

20 grams of shallots, diced

50 grams of peanuts

50 grams of spring onions, cut into rings

50 grams of bean sprouts

50 grams of spinach

100 grams of vine tomatoes, diced

150 grams of mushrooms, quartered

200 grams of ramen

1 liter of water

½ bunch of coriander, cut into small pieces

1 red chili, cut into thin strips

preparation

1   Heat the coconut oil in a saucepan and fry the mushrooms and shallots in it. Take both out of the saucepan, set them aside and steam the spring onions and tomatoes in the frying fat instead. Add the chili and fry it, then rub the whole thing off with the water.

2   Put the ramen in the pot, add the fried vegetables, spinach and sprouts and let everything simmer for 5 minutes.

3   Spread the dish in bowls and serve garnished with the peanuts and coriander.

www.ingramcontent.com/pod-product-compliance
Lightning Source LLC
Chambersburg PA
CBHW071111030426
42336CB00013BA/2035